QUICK AND

KETO

A Careful Selection of Delicious, Healthy
Low-Carb Recipes for Busy People

Written by

Sam Gallo

1

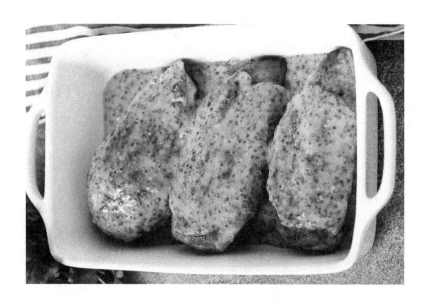

3

Table of Contents

Introduction

Want to follow a ketogenic diet but not sure where to start? Struggling with finding delicious and tummy-filling recipes when going "against the grains"? Do not worry! In this book you will find mouth-watering delights for any occasion and any eater, you will not believe that these recipes will help you restore your health and slim down your body.

Successfully practiced for more than nine decades, the ketogenic diet hs proven to be the ultimate long-term diet for any person. The restriction list may frighten many, but the truth is, this diet is super adaptable, and the food combinations and tasty meals are pretty endless.

Most people believe that our bodies are designed to run on carbohydrates. We think that ingesting carbohydrates is the only way to provide our bodies with the energy they need to function normally. However, what many people don't know is that carbohydrates are not the only source of fuel our bodies can use. Our bodies can also use fat as an energy source! When we decide to ditch carbs and provide our bodies with more fat, then we've begun our journey into the ketogenic diet, and this cookbook will be the guide you need to make your journey simple and enjoyable...let's start!

Breakfast recipes

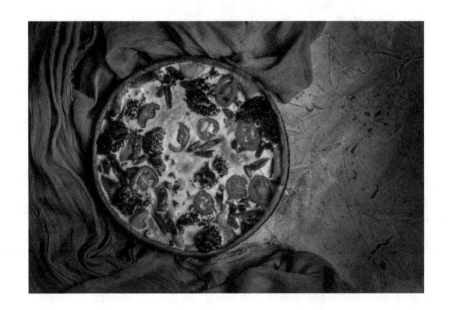

Quick Breakfast Porridge

Ingredients for 2 servings

½ tsp vanilla extract

2 tbsp chia seeds

4 tbsp hemp seeds

2 tbsp flaxseed meal

4 tbsp almond meal

4 tbsp shredded coconut

¼ tsp granulated stevia

2 tbsp walnuts, chopped

Directions and Total Time: approx. 10 minutes

Put chia seeds, hemp seeds, flaxseed meal, almond meal, granulated stevia, and shredded coconut in a nonstick saucepan and pour over ½ cup water. Simmer, stirring occasionally for about 3-4 minutes. Stir in vanilla. Sprinkle with chopped walnuts and serve warm.

Per serving: Cal 334; Net Carbs 1.5g; Fat 29g; Protein 15g

Mint Chocolate Protein Shake

Ingredients for 4 servings

3 cups flax milk, chilled

3 tsp cocoa powder

1 avocado, sliced

1 cup coconut milk, chilled

4 mint leaves

3 tbsp erythritol

1 scoop protein powder

Whipping cream for topping

Directions and Total Time: approx. 5 minutes

Combine flax milk, cocoa powder, avocado, coconut milk, erythritol, and protein powder into the smoothie maker and blend for 1 minute to smooth. Pour into serving cups, add some whipping cream on top, and garnish with mint.

Per serving: Cal 123; Net Carbs 4g; Fat 4.5g; Protein 15g

Zucchini Quiche with Pancetta Breakfast

Ingredients for 4 servings

2 medium zucchinis, diced

6 pancetta slices

4 eggs

1 tbsp olive oil

1 yellow onion, chopped

1 tbsp cilantro, chopped

Directions and Total Time: approx. 25 minutes

Warm olive oil in a skillet over medium heat. Place in the pancetta in a skillet and cook for 5 minutes, until crispy; reserve. Stir-fry the onion in the same skillet for 3 minutes. Add in zucchini and cook for 10 more minutes. Transfer to a plate. Fry the eggs into the same skillet. Top the zucchini mixture with pancetta, fried eggs, and cilantro.

Per serving: Cal 423; Net Carbs: 6g; Fat: 35g; Protein: 17g

Bok Choy Pumpkin Omelet with Sausage

Ingredients for 2 servings

2 eggs

1 cup bok choy, chopped

4 oz sausage, chopped

4 tbsp cotija cheese

4 oz pumpkin puree

1 tbsp olive oil

Directions and Total Time: approx. 10 minutes

Whisk eggs in a bowl. Stir in bok choy, cotija cheese, and pumpkin puree. Heat olive oil in a pan over medium heat and add sausage; cook for 5 minutes, stirring often.

Pour in eggs. Cook for 2 minutes or until the eggs are cooked. Fold in half and serve hot.

Per serving: Cal 558; Net Carbs 7.5g; Fat 52g; Protein 32g

Cauliflower & Ham Baked Eggs

Ingredients for 4 servings

2 heads cauliflower, cut into a small florets

2 bell peppers, chopped

¼ cup chopped ham

2 tsp ghee

1 tsp dried oregano

Salt and black pepper to taste

8 fresh eggs

Directions and Total Time: approx. 25 minutes

Preheat oven to 425 F. Melt ghee in a pan over medium heat and cook the ham, stirring frequently, about 3 minutes. Arrange cauliflower, bell peppers, and ham on a foil-lined baking sheet. Season with salt, oregano, and pepper. Bake for 10 minutes. Remove, create 8 indentations with a spoon, and crack an egg into each one. Return to the oven and continue baking for 7 more minutes. Serve warm.

Per serving: Cal 344; Net Carbs 4.2g; Fat 28g; Protein 11g

Butternut Squash & Zucchini Loaf Cake

Ingredients for 4 servings

5 large eggs

½ cup sour cream

1 cup butternut squash, grated

1 zucchini, grated

⅓ cup coconut flour

1 tbsp olive oil

¾ tsp baking powder

1 tbsp cinnamon powder

½ tsp salt

1 tsp white wine vinegar

½ tsp nutmeg powder

Directions and Total Time: approx. 70 minutes

Preheat oven to 360 F. Line a loaf pan with baking parchment. In a bowl, put coconut flour, baking powder, cinnamon powder, salt, and nutmeg. In a separate bowl, whisk eggs, olive oil, sour cream, and vinegar until combined. Add butternut squash and zucchini. Fold the dry mixture into the wet mixture. Pour the batter into the loaf pan and bake for 55 minutes. Let cool before slicing.

Per serving: Cal 186; Net Carbs 7.5g; Fat 12g; Protein 9.5g

Creamy Avocado Drink

Ingredients for 4 servings

4 avocados, halved and pitted

4 tbsp swerve sugar

¼ cup cold almond milk

1 tsp vanilla extract

1 tbsp cold heavy cream

Directions and Total Time: approx. 5 minutes

In a blender, add avocado, swerve sugar, milk, vanilla extract, and heavy cream. Process until smooth. Pour the mixture into 2 glasses, garnish with strawberries, and serve.

Per serving: Cal 388; Net Carbs 2.1g, Fat 32g, Protein 6.9g

Sausage & Grana Padano Egg Muffins

Ingredients for 3 servings

6 eggs, separated into yolks and whites

1 tsp butter, melted

½ tsp dried rosemary

1 cup Grana Padano, grated

3 beef sausages, chopped

Directions and Total Time: approx. 25 minutes

Set oven to 420 F. Lightly grease a muffin pan with the melted butter. Use an electric mixer to beat the egg whites until there is a formation of stiff peaks. Add in sausages, cheese, and seasonings. Pour into muffin cups and bake for 15 minutes. Place one egg yolk into each cup. Bake for an additional of 4 minutes. Let cool before serving.

Per serving: Cal 423; Net Carbs: 2g; Fat: 34g; Protein: 26g

Starter and Salad

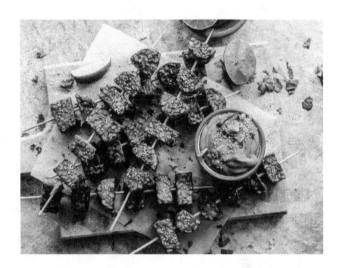

Caper & Artichoke Salad

Ingredients for 4 servings

¼ cup pitted green olives, sliced

6 baby artichokes

¼ cup cherry peppers, halved

¼ cup olive oil

¼ tsp lemon zest

2 tsp balsamic vinegar

1 tbsp chopped dill

Salt and black pepper to taste

1 tbsp capers

¼ tsp capers

Directions and Total Time: approx. 35 minutes

Trim and halve the artichokes and put in a pot over medium heat and cover with salted water. Bring to a boil, lower the heat, and let simmer for 20 minutes until tender. Combine the rest of the ingredients, except for olives in a bowl. Drain and plate the artichokes. Pour the prepared mixture over and toss to combine. Serve topped with olives.

Per serving: Cal 170; Net Carbs 5g; Fat 13g; Protein 1g

Cheddar & Chive Soufflés

Ingredients for 4 servings

½ cup almond flour

Salt to taste

1 tsp ground mustard

½ tsp black pepper

½ tsp arrowroot starch

¼ tsp cayenne pepper

¾ cup heavy cream

2 cups grated cheddar cheese

¼ cup chopped fresh chives

6 eggs, separated yolks and whites

¼ tsp cream of tartar

Directions and Total Time: approx. 30 minutes

Preheat oven to 350 F. Grease 8 ramekins with melted butter and arrange the ramekins on a large cookie sheet. In a bowl, whisk flour, salt, mustard, black pepper, arrowroot starch and cayenne pepper. Whisk in heavy cream until well combined. Mix in cheddar cheese, chives, and egg yolks until well combined. In a large, clean bowl, beat the egg whites, cream of tartar and salt until stiff peaks form and glossy.

Carefully fold this mixture into the cheese mix until well incorporated. Divide the mixture into the ramekins, place the cookie sheet in the oven and bake for

25 minutes or until the soufflés have risen by an inch or 2 above the rim and are golden brown. Remove and serve.

Per serving: Cal 460; Net Carbs 2g, Fat 38g, Protein 26g

Spinach Muffins

Ingredients for 4 servings

1 large egg, separated into egg white and yolk

½ tsp salted butter

1/8 tsp cream of tartar

2 tbsp heavy cream

2 tbsp almond flour

1/8 tsp arrowroot starch

Salt and black pepper to taste

1/8 tsp onion powder

2 tbsp grated mozzarella

¼ oz chopped spinach

Directions and Total Time: approx. 35 minutes

Preheat oven to 350 F. Grease 8 ramekins with butter and arrange them on a large cookie sheet. Remove to the fridge. Whip the egg white and cream of tartar using an electric mixer until stiff peaks forms. In another bowl, whisk the egg yolk and heavy cream until pale yellow and slightly thickened. Add almond flour, arrowroot starch, salt, pepper, and onion powder. Mix smoothly and fold in mozzarella cheese and spinach.

Mix one-third of the egg white mixture into the spinach mix until well incorporated. Add another third of the egg white mixture, mix again, and then add the last bit of the egg white mixture. Once well-mixed, divide the batter between the ramekins. Bake for 25 minutes or until golden brown on top, crisp around the edges, and tender inside.

Per serving: Cal 78; Net Carbs 2.4g, Fat 6.3g, Protein 3.4g

Cheese & Bacon Cups

Ingredients for 4 servings

4 eggs, separated into egg whites and egg yolks

2 tbsp butter

2 tbsp almond flour

1 cup heavy cream

1 ½ cups shredded Parmesan

4 oz bacon, chopped, cooked

Directions and Total Time: approx. 50 minutes

Preheat oven to 350 F. Butter 4 ramekins with some butter. Place the ramekins on a cookie sheet and set aside. Melt the remaining butter over medium heat and mix in 1 tbsp of almond flour until well combined. Whisk in heavy cream and bring to a boil with frequent stirring. Mix in almond flour until well combined. Turn the heat off and let cool for 3 minutes. Whisk in eggs yolks one after another until well combined and then, mix in Parmesan cheese. Beat the egg whites until stiff peaks form. Slowly fold this mixture into the egg yolk mix until with combined. Divide the mixture between the ramekins, top with bacon, and bake for 35 minutes or until slight risen above the rim of the ramekins and golden brown. Serve chilled.

Per serving: Cal 437; Net Carbs 4.8g, Fat 47g, Protein 21g

Lobster Roll Salad

Ingredients for 4 servings

5 cups cauliflower florets

⅓ cup diced celery

½ cup sliced black olives

2 cups cooked jumbo shrimp

1 tbsp dill, chopped

½ cup mayonnaise

1 tsp apple cider vinegar

¼ tsp celery seeds

2 tbsp lemon juice

2 tsp swerve sweetener

Directions and Total Time: approx. 1 hour 10 minutes

Combine cauliflower, celery, shrimp, olives, and dill in a large bowl. Whisk mayonnaise, vinegar, celery seeds, swerve sweetener, and lemon juice in another bowl. Pour the dressing over the salad and toss to combine. Refrigerate for 1 hour. Serve topped with olives.

Per serving: Cal 182; Net Carbs 2g; Fat 15g; Protein 12g

Bacon & Avocado Salad

Ingredients for 4 servings

2 avocados, 1 chopped and 1 sliced

4 cooked bacon slices, crumbled

1 spring onion, sliced

2 cups spinach, chopped

1 lettuce head, chopped

2 hard-boiled eggs, chopped

3 tbsp olive oil

1 tsp Dijon mustard

1 tbsp apple cider vinegar

Salt and black pepper to taste

Directions and Total Time: approx. 20 minutes

Combine spinach, lettuce, eggs, chopped avocado, and spring onion in a large bowl. Whisk the olive oil, mustard, and vinegar in another bowl. Pour the dressing over. Toss to combine. Serve topped with sliced avocado and bacon.

Per serving: Cal 350; Net Carbs 3.4g; Fat 33g; Protein 7g

Soup and stews

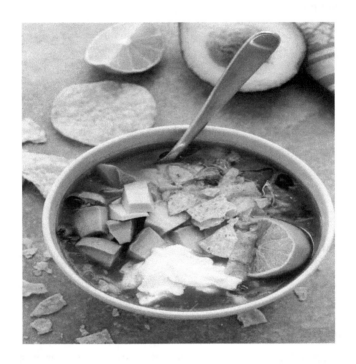

Coconut Cream Soup

Ingredients for 4 servings

1 small head cauliflower, cut into florets

2 tbsp coconut oil

½ lb celery root, chopped

1 garlic clove, minced

1 white onion, sliced

¼ cup dill, roughly chopped

1 tsp cumin powder

¼ tsp nutmeg powder

4 cups vegetable stock

2 tbsp butter

Juice from 1 lemon

¼ cup coconut cream

Salt and black pepper to taste

Directions and Total Time: approx. 25 minutes

Warm coconut oil in a pot over medium heat and sauté celery root, garlic, and onion until fragrant and soft, about 5 minutes. Stir in dill, cumin, and nutmeg and fry further for 1 minute. Mix in cauli florets and vegetable stock. Bring the soup to a boil for 15 minutes. Turn the heat off. Add in butter and lemon juice. Puree the ingredients with an immersion blender until smooth. Mix in coconut cream and season to taste. Spoon into bowls and serve warm.

Mixed Mushroom Soup

Ingredients for 4 servings

5 oz white button mushrooms, chopped

5 oz cremini mushrooms, chopped

5 oz shiitake mushrooms, chopped

1 vegetable stock cube, crushed

4 oz unsalted butter

1 small onion, finely chopped

1 clove garlic, minced

½ lb celery root, chopped

½ tsp dried rosemary

1 tbsp plain vinegar

1 cup coconut cream

6 leaves basil, chopped

Directions and Total Time: approx. 35 minutes

Melt butter in a saucepan over medium heat. Sauté onion, garlic, mushrooms, and celery until fragrant, 6 minutes.

Reserve some mushrooms for garnishing. Add in rosemary, 4 cups of water, stock cube, and vinegar. Stir and bring to a boil; reduce the heat and simmer for 20 minutes. Mix in coconut cream and puree. Garnish with the reserved mushrooms and basil and serve.

Per serving: Cal 506; Fat 46g; Net Carbs 12g; Protein 8g

Broccoli & Fennel Soup

Ingredients for 4 servings

1 fennel bulb, chopped

10 oz broccoli, cut into florets

4 cups vegetable stock

Salt and black pepper to taste

1 garlic clove

1 cup cream cheese

2 tbsp butter

½ cup chopped fresh oregano

Directions and Total Time: approx. 25 minutes

Put fennel, broccoli, and garlic in a pot over medium heat and pour in the vegetable stock. Bring to a boil and simmer until the vegetables are soft, about 10 minutes. Season with salt and pepper. Pour in cream cheese, butter, and oregano. Puree the ingredients with an immersion blender until smooth. Serve with cheese crackers.

Per serving: Cal 510; Fat 44g; Net Carbs 7g; Protein 16g

Parsnip–Tomato Soup

Ingredients for 4 servings

1 tbsp butter

1 tbsp olive oil

1 large red onion, chopped

4 garlic cloves, minced

6 red bell peppers, sliced

1 daikon radish, chopped

2 parsnips, chopped

3 cups chopped tomatoes

4 cups vegetable stock

3 cups coconut milk

2 cups chopped walnuts

1 cup grated Parmesan cheese

Directions and Total Time: approx. 40 minutes

Heat butter and olive oil in a pot over medium heat and sauté onion and garlic for 3 minutes. Stir in bell peppers, daikon radish, and parsnips; cook for 10 minutes. Pour in tomatoes and vegetable stock; simmer for 20 minutes. Puree the soup with an immersion blender. Mix in coconut milk. Garnish with walnuts and Parmesan cheese to serve.

Per serving: Cal 955; Net Carbs 4g; Fat 86g, Protein 19.1g

Herby Cheese & Bacon Soup

Ingredients for 4 servings

1 tbsp olive oil

6 slices bacon, chopped

1 tbsp butter

1 small white onion, chopped

3 garlic cloves, minced

2 tbsp finely chopped thyme

1 tbsp chopped fresh tarragon

1 tbsp chopped fresh oregano

2 cups cubed parsnips

3 ½ cups vegetable broth

Salt and black pepper to taste

1 cup almond milk

1 cup grated cheddar cheese

2 tbsp chopped scallions

Directions and Total Time: approx. 25 minutes

Heat olive oil in a saucepan over medium heat and fry bacon until browned and crunchy, 5 minutes; set aside. Melt butter in the saucepan and sauté onion, garlic, thyme, tarragon, and oregano for 3 minutes. Add in the parsnips, season with salt and pepper, and cook for 15 minutes until the parsnips soften. Using an immersion blender, process the soup until smooth. Stir in almond milk and cheddar cheese and simmer with continuous stirring until the cheese melts. Top with bacon and scallions and serve.

Per serving: Cal 775; Net Carbs 6.5g; Fat 57g, Protein 18g

Lunch and dinner

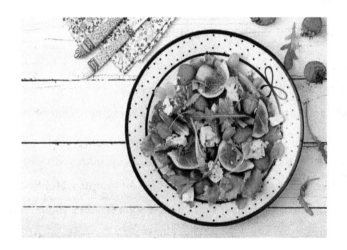

Cheesy Muffins with Ajillo Mushrooms

Ingredients for 6 servings

1 ½ cups heavy cream

5 ounces mascarpone cheese

3 eggs, beaten

1 tbsp butter, softened

2 cups mushrooms, chopped

2 garlic cloves, minced

Directions and Total Time: approx. 45 minutes

Preheat oven to 320 F. Insert 6 ramekins into a large pan. Add in boiling water up to 1-inch depth. In a pan over medium heat, warm heavy cream. Set heat to low and stir in mascarpone cheese; cook until melted. Place beaten eggs in a bowl and place in 3 tbsp of the hot cream mixture; mix well. Place the mixture back to the pan with hot cream/cheese mixture. Sprinkle with pepper and salt. Ladle the mixture into the ramekins. Bake for 40 minutes. Melt butter in a pan and add garlic and mushrooms; sauté for 5-6 minutes. Top the muffins with the mushrooms.

Per serving: Cal 263; Net Carbs: 6g; Fat: 22g; Protein: 10g

Easy Lamb Kebabs

Ingredients for 4 servings

1 pound ground lamb

¼ tsp cinnamon

1 egg

1 grated onion

Salt and black pepper to taste

2 tbsp mint, chopped

Directions and Total Time: approx. 20 minutes

Place all ingredients in a bowl; mix to combine. Divide the meat into 4 pieces. Shape all of the meat portions around previously-soaked skewers. Preheat grill to medium heat. Grill the kebabs for 5 minutes per side. Serve warm.

Per serving: Cal 467; Net Carbs 3.2g; Fat 37g; Protein 27g

Basic Keto Pizza Dough

Ingredients for 8 servings

3 cups almond flour

3 tbsp ghee

¼ tsp salt

3 large eggs

Directions and Total Time: approx. 10 minutes

Preheat oven to 350 F. In a bowl, mix almond flour, ghee, salt, and eggs until a dough forms. Mold the dough into a ball and place between 2 wide pieces of parchment paper on a flat surface. Use a pin roll it out into a circle of a quarter-inch thickness. Slide the dough into the pizza pan and remove the parchment papers. Bake for 20 minutes. Decorate with your favorite topping and bake further.

Per serving: Cal 151; Net Carbs: 2g; Fat: 11g; Protein: 7g

Tomato Pizza with Strawberries

Ingredients for 4 servings

3 cups shredded mozzarella

2 tbsp cream cheese, softened

¾ cup almond flour

2 tbsp almond meal

1 celery stalk, chopped

1 tomato, chopped

1 tbsp olive oil

2 tbsp balsamic vinegar

1 cup strawberries, halved

1 tbsp chopped mint leaves

Directions and Total Time: approx. 35 minutes

Preheat oven to 390 F. Line a pizza pan with parchment paper. Microwave 2 cups of mozzarella cheese and cream cheese for 1 minute. Remove and mix in almond flour and almond meal. Spread the mixture on the pizza pan and bake for 10 minutes. Spread remaining mozzarella cheese on the crust. In a bowl, toss celery, tomato, olive oil, and balsamic vinegar. Spoon the mixture onto the mozzarella cheese and arrange the strawberries on top. Top with mint leaves. Bake for 15 minutes. Serve sliced.

Per serving: Cal 306; Net Carbs 4g; Fats 11g; Protein 28g

Cheesy Brussels Sprouts Salad

Ingredients for 6 servings

2 lb Brussels sprouts, halved

3 tbsp olive oil

Salt and black pepper to taste

2 ½ tbsp balsamic vinegar

¼ red cabbage, shredded

1 tbsp Dijon mustard

1 cup Parmesan, grated

2 tbsp pumpkin seeds, toasted

Directions and Total Time: approx. 35 minutes

Preheat oven to 400 F. Line a baking sheet with foil. Toss brussels sprouts with olive oil, salt, pepper, and balsamic vinegar in a bowl and spread on the baking sheet. Bake for 20-25 minutes. Transfer to a salad bowl and mix in red cabbage, mustard, and half of the cheese. Sprinkle with the remaining cheese and pumpkin seeds and serve.

Per serving: Cal 210; Net Carbs 6g; Fat 18g; Protein 4g

Tomato Bites with Vegan Cheese Topping

Ingredients for 6 servings

2 spring onions, chopped

5 tomatoes, sliced

¼ cup olive oil

1 tbsp seasoning mix

For vegan cheese

½ cup pepitas seeds

1 tbsp nutritional yeast

Salt and black pepper, to taste

1 tsp garlic puree

Directions and Total Time: approx. 15 minutes

Drizzle tomatoes with olive oil. Preheat oven to 400 F. In a food processor, add all vegan cheese ingredients and pulse until the desired consistency is attained. Combine vegan cheese and seasoning mix. Toss in the tomato slices to coat. Set tomato slices on a baking pan and bake for 10 minutes. Top with spring onions and serve.

Per serving: Cal 161; Net Carbs: 7g; Fat: 14g; Protein: 5g

Kale & Mushroom Pierogis

Ingredients for 4 servings

7 tbsp butter

2 garlic cloves, minced

1 small red onion, chopped

3 oz bella mushrooms, sliced

2 oz fresh kale

Salt and black pepper to taste

½ cup cream cheese

2 cups Parmesan, grated

1 tbsp flax seed powder

½ cup almond flour

4 tbsp coconut flour

1 tsp baking powder

Directions and Total Time: approx. 45 minutes

Melt 2 tbsp of butter in a skillet and sauté garlic, red onion, mushrooms, and kale for 5 minutes. Season with salt and pepper and reduce the heat to low. Stir in cream cheese and ½ cup of Parmesan cheese; simmer for 1 minute. Set aside to cool. In a bowl, mix flax seed powder with 3 tbsp water and allow sitting for 5 minutes. In a another bowl, combine almond and coconut flours, salt, and baking powder. Put a pan over low heat and melt the remaining Parmesan cheese and butter. Turn the heat off.

Pour the flax egg in the cream mixture, continue stirring, while adding the flour mixture until a firm dough forms. Mold the dough into balls, place on a chopping board, and use a rolling pin to flatten each into ½ inch thin round piece. Spread a generous amount of stuffing on one-half of each dough, fold over the filling, and seal the dough with fingers. Brush with oil and bake for 20 minutes at 380 F.

Per serving: Cal 540; Net Carbs 6g; Fat 47g; Protein 18g

Salami Cauliflower Pizza

Ingredients for 4 servings

2 cups grated mozzarella

4 cups cauliflower rice

1 tbsp dried thyme

¼ cup tomato sauce

4 oz salami slices

Directions and Total Time: approx. 40 minutes

Preheat oven to 390 F. Microwave cauliflower rice mixed with 1 tbsp of water for 1 minute. Remove and mix in 1 cup of the mozzarella cheese and thyme.

Pour the mixture into a greased baking dish, spread out and bake for 5 minutes. Remove the dish and spread the tomato sauce on top. Scatter remaining mozzarella cheese on the sauce and then arrange salami slices on top. Bake for 15 minutes.

Per serving: Cal 276; Net Carbs 2g; Fats 15g; Protein 20g

Baked Cheese & Cauliflower

Ingredients for 4 servings

1 head cauliflower, cut into florets

¼ cup butter, cubed

2 tbsp melted butter

1 white onion, chopped

¼ almond milk

½ cup almond flour

1 ½ cups grated Colby cheese

Directions and Total Time: approx. 30 minutes

Preheat oven to 350 F. Microwave the cauli florets for 4-5 minutes. Melt the butter cubes in a saucepan and sauté onion for 3 minutes. Add in cauliflower, season with salt and pepper, and mix in almond milk. Simmer for 3 minutes. Mix the remaining melted butter with almond flour. Stir into the cauliflower as well as half of the cheese. Sprinkle the top with the remaining cheese and bake for 10 minutes. Plate the bake and serve with arugula salad.

Per serving: Cal 215; Net Carbs 4g; Fat 15g; Protein 12g

Poultry

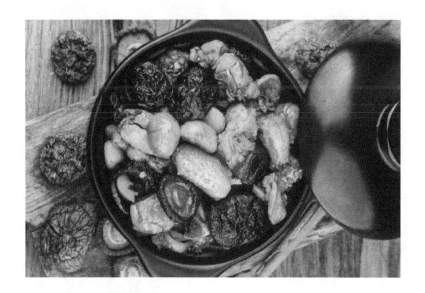

Celery & Radish Chicken Casserole

Ingredients for 4 servings

½ lemon, juiced

3 tbsp basil pesto

¾ cup heavy cream

½ cup cream cheese, softened

3 tbsp butter

2 lb chicken breasts, cubed

1 celery, chopped

¼ cup chopped tomatoes

1 lb radishes, sliced

½ cup shredded Pepper Jack

Directions and Total Time: approx. 50 minutes

Preheat oven to 400 F. In a bowl, combine lemon juice, pesto, heavy cream, and cream cheese; set aside. Melt butter in a skillet and cook the chicken cook until no longer pink, 8 minutes. Transfer to a greased casserole and spread the pesto mixture on top. Top with celery, tomatoes, and radishes. Sprinkle Pepper Jack cheese on top and bake for 30 minutes or until the cheese melts and golden brown on top. Serve with braised green beans.

Per serving: Cal 667; Net Carbs 0.8g; Fat 47g; Protein 51g

Broccoli & Cheese Chicken Sausage

Ingredients for 4 servings

2 tbsp salted butter

4 links chicken sausages, sliced

3 cups broccoli florets

4 garlic cloves, minced

½ cup tomato sauce

¼ cup red wine

½ tsp red pepper flakes

3 cups chopped kale

½ cup Pecorino Romano

Salt and black pepper to taste

Directions and Total Time: approx. 30 minutes

Melt half of the butter in a wok and fry the sausages until brown, 5 minutes; set aside. Melt the remaining butter in the wok and sauté broccoli for 5 minutes. Mix in garlic and cook for 3 minutes, then pour in tomato sauce, red wine, red pepper flakes, and season with salt and pepper. Cover the lid and cook for 10 minutes or until the tomato sauce reduces by one-third. Return the sausages to the pan and heat for 1 minute. Stir in kale to wilt. Spoon onto a platter and sprinkle with Pecorino Romano cheese. Serve.

Per serving: Cal 263; Net Carbs 7.1g; Fat 17g; Protein 15g

Smoked Chicken Tart with Baby Kale

Ingredients for 4 servings

1 cup shredded provolone cheese

1 lb ground chicken

2 cups powdered Parmesan

¼ tsp onion powder

¼ tsp garlic powder

½ cup tomato sauce

1 tsp white winw vinegar

½ tsp liquid smoke

¼ cup baby kale, chopped

Directions and Total Time: approx. 30 minutes

Preheat oven to 400 F. Line a pizza pan with parchment paper and grease with cooking spray. In a bowl, combine chicken and Parmesan cheese. Spread the mixture on the pan to fit. Bake for 15 minutes until the chicken cooks. In a bowl, mix onion and garlic powder, tomato sauce, white wine vinegar, and liquid smoke. Remove the meat crust from the oven and spread tomato mixture on top. Add kale and sprinkle with provolone cheese. Bake for 7 minutes or until the cheese melts. Slice and serve warm.

Per serving: Cal 517; Net Carbs 16g; Fat 28g; Protein 46g

Melt-In-The-Middle Chicken Meatballs

Ingredients for 4 servings

2 tbsp olive oil

1 large egg

1 pound ground chicken

1 cup celery, chopped

2 tbsp pork rinds, crushed

2 garlic cloves, minced

2 shallots, chopped

1 tbsp dried oregano

2 tbsp fresh parsley, chopped

1 cup Pecorino cheese, grated

Directions and Total Time: approx. 20 minutes

Put ground chicken, egg, shallots, garlic, celery, oregano, parsley, black pepper, and salt in a bowl and mix to combine. Form meatballs from the mixture. Lay the pork rinds on a large plate and roll the meatballs in them. Fry the meatballs in warm olive oil over medium heat on all sides until lightly golden, about 5-6 minutes and transfer to a baking dish. Scatter the grated cheese over and bake for 5 minutes or until the cheese melts. Serve warm.

Per serving: Cal 466; Net Carbs 2.7g; Fat 35g; Protein 32g

Parsley Chicken & Cauliflower Stir-Fry

Ingredients for 4 servings

1 large head cauliflower, cut into florets

2 tbsp olive oil

2 chicken breasts, sliced

1 red bell pepper, diced

1 yellow bell pepper, diced

3 tbsp chicken broth

2 tbsp chopped parsley

Directions and Total Time: approx. 30 minutes

Heat olive oil in a skillet and brown the chicken until brown on all sides, 8 minutes. Transfer to a plate. Pour bell peppers into the pan and sauté until softened, 5 minutes. Add in cauliflower and chicken broth and mix. Cover the pan and cook for 5 minutes or until cauliflower is tender. Mix in chicken and parsley. Serve immediately.

Per serving: Cal 345; Net Carbs 3.5g; Fat 21g; Protein 32g

Greek-Style Chicken Drumsticks

Ingredients for 4 servings

5 kaffir lime leaves

1 tbsp cumin powder

1 tbsp ginger powder

1 cup Greek yogurt

2 lb chicken drumsticks

Salt and black pepper to taste

1 tbsp olive oil

2 limes, juiced

Directions and Total Time: approx. 35 min + chilling time

In a bowl, combine kaffir leaves, cumin, ginger, and Greek yogurt. Add in chicken, salt, and pepper and mix to coat. Cover the bowl with plastic wrap and marinate in the fridge for 3 hours. Preheat oven to 350 F. Arrange chicken on a greased baking sheet. Drizzle with olive oil and lime juice, cover with aluminum foil, and bake for 20-25 minutes. Remove foil, turn broiler on, and brown the chicken for 10 minutes. Serve with red cabbage slaw.

Per serving: Cal 463; Net Carbs 6.1g; Fat 27g; Protein 44g

Lettuce Chicken Fajita Bowl with Cilantro

Ingredients for 4 servings

1½ lb boneless chicken breasts, cut into strips

½ cup shredded Mexican cheese blend

2 tbsp olive oil

Salt and black pepper to taste

2 tbsp Tex-Mex seasoning

1 iceberg lettuce, chopped

2 tomatoes, and chopped

2 avocados, chopped

1 green bell pepper, sliced

1 yellow onion, thinly sliced

4 tbsp fresh cilantro leaves

1 cup crème fraiche

Directions and Total Time: approx. 20 minutes

Heat olive oil in a skillet, season the chicken with salt, pepper, and Tex-Mex seasoning, and fry until golden, 10 minutes; transfer to a plate. Divide lettuce into 4 bowls, share the chicken on top, and add tomatoes, avocados, bell pepper, onion, cilantro, and Mexican cheese. Top with dollops of crème fraiche and serve with low carb tortillas.

Per serving: Cal 626; Net Carbs 4.5g; Fat 42g; Protein 47g

Chili Pulled Chicken with Avocado

Ingredients for 4 servings

1 white onion, finely chopped

¼ cup chicken stock

3 tbsp coconut oil

3 tbsp tamari sauce

3 tbsp chili pepper

1 tbsp red wine vinegar

Salt and black pepper to taste

2 lb boneless chicken thighs

1 avocado, halved and pitted

½ lemon, juiced

Directions and Total Time: approx. 2 hours 30 minutes

In a pot, combine onion, stock, coconut oil, tamari sauce, chili, vinegar, salt, and pepper. Add in thighs, close the lid, and cook over low heat for 2 hours. Scoop avocado pulp into a bowl, add lemon juice, and mash the avocado into a puree; set aside. When the chicken is ready, open the lid and use two forks to shred it. Cook further for 15 minutes. Turn the heat off and mix in avocado. Serve warm.

Per serving: Cal 710; Net Carbs 4g; Fat 56g; Protein 40g

Parmesan Chicken & Broccoli Casserole

Ingredients for 4 servings

5 tbsp butter

1 small white onion, chopped

2 garlic cloves, minced

1 lb ground chicken

1 lb broccoli rabe, chopped

1 cup grated Parmesan cheese

Directions and Total Time: approx. 40 minutes

Preheat oven to 350 F. Melt butter in a skillet and sauté onion and garlic for 3 minutes. Put in chicken and cook until no longer pink, 8 minutes. Add chicken and broccoli rabe to a greased baking dish and mix evenly. Top with butter from the skillet and sprinkle Parmesan cheese on top. Bake for 20 minutes until the cheese melts. Serve.

Per serving: Cal 429; Net Carbs 4.3g; Fat 31g; Protein 31g

Beef

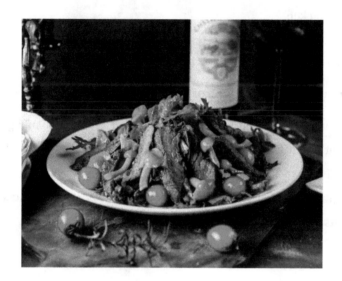

Beef Steak Fajitas

Ingredients for 4 servings

2 lb flank steak, cut in halves

2 tbsp Adobo seasoning

2 tbsp olive oil

2 large white onion, chopped

1 cup sliced bell peppers

12 zero carb tortillas

Directions and Total Time: approx. 20 min + marunating time

Rub the steak with adobo seasoning and marinate in the fridge for 1 hour. Preheat grill and cook steak for 6 minutes on each side, flipping once. Remove from heat and wrap in foil and let sit for 10 minutes. Heat olive oil in a skillet and sauté onion and bell peppers for 5 minutes. Cut steak against the grain into strips and share on the tortillas. Top with vegetables and serve.

Per serving: Cal 348, Net Carbs 5g, Fat 25g, Protein 18g

Garlicky Beef with Creamy Curry Sauce

Ingredients for 4 servings

2 tbsp ghee

4 large rib-eye steak

2 garlic cloves, minced

½ cup chopped brown onion

1 green bell pepper, sliced

1 red bell pepper, sliced

2 long red chilies, sliced

1 cup beef stock

1 cup coconut milk

1 tbsp Thai green curry paste

1 lime, juiced

2 tbsp chopped cilantro

Directions and Total Time: approx. 40 minutes

Melt the 1 tbsp of ghee in a pan over medium heat and cook the beef for 3 minutes on each side. Remove to a plate. Add the remaining ghee to the skillet and sauté garlic and onion for 3 minutes. Stir-fry in bell peppers and red chili until softened, 5 minutes. Pour in beef stock, coconut milk, curry paste, and lime juice. Let simmer for 4 minutes. Put the beef back into the sauce, cook for 10 minutes, and transfer the pan to the oven. Cook further under the broiler for 5 minutes. Garnish with cilantro and serve with cauliflower rice.

Bacon-Wrapped Beef Hot Dogs

Ingredients for 4 servings

8 large beef hot dogs

½ cup grated Gruyere cheese

16 slices bacon

1 tsp onion powder

1 tsp garlic powder

Salt and black pepper to taste

Directions and Total Time: approx. 45 minutes

Preheat oven to 400 F. Cut a slit in the middle of each hot dog and stuff evenly with cheese. Wrap each hot dog with 2 bacon slices and secure with toothpicks. Season with onion and garlic powders, salt, and pepper. Place the hot dogs in the middle rack of the oven and slide in the cookie sheet beneath the rack to catch dripping grease. Cook for 15 minutes until the bacon browns and crisps. Serve.

Per serving: Cal 758; Net Carbs 4g; Fat 56g; Protein 37g

Walnut Beef Skillet with Brussels Sprouts

Ingredients for 4 servings

¼ cup toasted walnuts, chopped

1 ½ cups Brussels sprouts, halved

2 tbsp avocado oil

1 garlic clove, minced

½ white onion, chopped

Salt and black pepper to taste

1 lb ground beef

1 bok choy, quartered

2 tbsp chopped scallions

1 tbsp black sesame seeds

Directions and Total Time: approx. 30 minutes

Heat 1 tbsp of avocado oil in a skillet over medium heat and sauté garlic and onion for 3 minutes. Stir in ground beef and cook until brown while breaking the lumps, 7 minutes. Pour in Brussels sprouts, bok choy, walnuts, scallions, and season with salt and black pepper. Sauté for 5 minutes. Serve with low carb bread.

Per serving: Cal 302; Net Carbs 3.1g; Fat 18g; Protein 29g

Sage Beef Meatloaf with Pecans

Ingredients for 4 servings

2 tbsp olive oil

1 white onion, finely chopped

1 ½ lb ground beef

½ cup coconut cream

½ cup shredded Parmesan

1 egg, lightly beaten

1 tbsp dried sage

4 tbsp toasted pecans, chopped

Salt and black pepper to taste

6 bacon slices

Directions and Total Time: approx. 45 minutes

Preheat oven to 400 F. Heat olive oil in a skillet and sauté the onion for 3 minutes. In a bowl, mix ground beef, onion, coconut cream, Parmesan cheese, egg, sage, pecans, salt, and pepper. Form into a loaf, wrap it with bacon slices, secure with toothpicks, and place on a greased baking sheet. Bake for 30 minutes. Serve sliced.

Per serving: Cal 617; Net Carbs 6.6g; Fat 43g; Protein 48g

Parsley Steak Bites with Shirataki Fettucine

Ingredients for 4 servings

2 (8 oz) packs shirataki fettuccine

1 lb thick-cut New York strip steaks, cut into 1-inch cubes

1 cup freshly grated Pecorino Romano cheese

4 tbsp butter

Salt and black pepper to taste

4 garlic cloves, minced

2 tbsp chopped fresh parsley

Directions and Total Time: approx. 30 minutes

Boil 2 cups of water in a pot. Strain the shirataki pasta and rinse well under hot running water. Allow proper draining and pour into the boiling water. Cook for 3 minutes and strain again. Place a dry skillet and stir-fry the shirataki pasta until visibly dry, 1-2 minutes; set aside. Melt butter in a skillet over medium heat, season the steaks with salt and pepper, and cook for 10 minutes. Stir in garlic and cook for 1 minute. Mix in parsley and shirataki; toss to coat. Top with the Pecorino Romano cheese and serve.

Per serving: Cal 422; Net Carbs 7g; Fats 22g; Protein 36g

Cabbage & Beef Bowl with Blue Cheese

Ingredients for 4 servings

2 tbsp butter

1 canon cabbage, shredded

1 tsp onion powder

1 tsp garlic powder

1 tsp dried oregano

1 tbsp red wine vinegar

1 ½ lb ground beef

1 cup coconut cream

¼ cup blue cheese

½ cup fresh parsley, chopped

Directions and Total Time: approx. 25 minutes

Melt butter in a deep skillet and sauté cabbage, onion and garlic powders, oregano, salt, pepper, and vinegar for 5 minutes; set aside. Add the beef to the skillet and cook until browned, frequently stirring and breaking the lumps, 10 minutes. Stir in coconut cream and blue cheese until the cheese melts, 3 minutes. Return the cabbage mixture and add parsley. Stir-fry for 2 minutes. Dish into serving bowls and serve with low carb bread.

Per serving: Cal 542; Net Carbs 4.2g; Fat 41g; Protein 41g

Beef Broccoli Curry

Ingredients for 6 servings

1 head broccoli, cut into florets

3 tbsp olive oil

1 ½ lb ground beef

1 tbsp ginger-garlic paste

1 tsp garam masala

1 (7 oz) can whole tomatoes

Salt and chili pepper to taste

Directions and Total Time: approx. 30 minutes

Heat olive oil in a saucepan over medium heat and add beef, ginger-garlic paste, garam masala. Cook for 5 minutes. Stir in tomatoes and broccoli, season with salt and chili pepper, and cook for 6 minutes.

Add ¼ cup of water and bring to a boil for 10 minutes or until the water has reduced by half. Spoon into serving bowls and serve.

Per serving: Cal 374, Net Carbs 2g, Fat 33g, Protein 22g

Pork

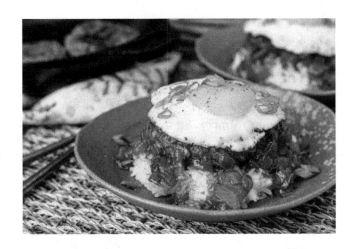

Tender Pork Chops with Basil & Beet Greens

Ingredients for 4 servings

2 cups chopped beetroot greens

2 tbsp balsamic vinegar

2 tsp freshly pureed garlic

2 tbsp freshly chopped basil

1 tbsp olive oil

4 pork chops

2 tbsp butter

Salt and black pepper to taste

Directions and Total Time: approx. 30 minutes

Preheat oven to 400 F. In a saucepan over low heat, add vinegar, garlic, salt, pepper, and basil. Cook until the mixture is syrupy. Heat olive oil in a skillet and sear pork on both sides for 8 minutes. Brush the vinegar glaze on the pork and bake for 8 minutes. Melt butter in another skillet and sauté beetroot greens for 5 minutes. Serve with pork.

Per serving: Cal 391; Net Carbs 0.8g; Fat 16g; Protein 40g

Cheddar Pork Burrito Bowl

Ingredients for 4 servings

1 tbsp butter

1 lb ground pork

½ cup beef broth

4 tbsp taco seasoning

Salt and black pepper to taste

½ cup sharp cheddar, shredded

½ cup sour cream

¼ cup sliced black olives

1 avocado, cubed

¼ cup tomatoes, diced

1 green onion, sliced

1 tbsp fresh cilantro, chopped

Directions and Total Time: approx. 30 minutes

Melt butter in a skillet over medium heat. Cook the ground pork until brown while breaking any lumps, 10 minutes. Mix in broth, taco seasoning, salt, and pepper; cook until most of the liquid evaporates, 5 minutes. Mix in cheddar cheese to melt. Spoon into a serving bowl and top with olives, avocado, tomatoes, green onion, and cilantro.

Per serving: Cal 386; Net Carbs 8.8g; Fat 23g; Protein 30g

Pork & Eggs with Brussels Sprouts

Ingredients for 4 servings

2 tbsp sesame oil

2 large eggs

2 garlic cloves, minced

½ tsp ginger puree

1 medium white onion, diced

1 lb ground pork

1 habanero pepper, chopped

1 lb Brussels sprouts, halved

3 tbsp coconut aminos

1 tbsp white wine vinegar

2 tbsp sesame seeds

Salt and black pepper to taste

Directions and Total Time: approx. 30 minutes

Heat 1 tbsp of sesame oil in a skillet and scramble the eggs until set, 1 minute; set aside. Heat remaining sesame oil in the same skillet and sauté garlic, ginger, and onion until soft and fragrant, 4 minutes. Add in ground pork and habanero pepper and season with salt and pepper. Cook for 10 minutes. Mix in Brussels sprouts, aminos, and wine vinegar and cook until the sprouts are tender. Stir in the eggs. Serve garnished with sesame seeds.

Per serving: Cal 295; Net Carbs 3.6g; Fat 16g; Protein 29g

Parmesan Pork Stuffed Mushrooms

Ingredients for 4 servings

12 portobello mushroom caps

2 tbsp butter

½ lb ground pork

1 tsp paprika

Salt and black pepper to taste

3 tbsp chives, finely chopped

7 oz cream cheese

¼ cup shredded Parmesan

Directions and Total Time: approx. 30 minutes

Preheat oven to 400 F. Melt butter in a skillet, add the ground pork, season with paprika, salt, and pepper and stir-fry until brown, 10 minutes. Mix in two-thirds of chives and cream cheese until evenly combined. Spoon the mixture into the mushroom caps and transfer them to a greased baking sheet. Top with the Parmesan cheese and bake until mushrooms turn golden and the cheese melts, 10 minutes. Garnish with the remaining chives and serve.

Per serving: Cal 299; Net Carbs 2.2g; Fat 23g; Protein 19g

Florentine-Style Pizza with Bacon

Ingredients for 4 servings

1 cup shredded provolone cheese

1 (7 oz) can sliced mushrooms, drained

10 eggs

1 tsp Italian seasoning

6 bacon slices

2/3 cup tomato sauce

2 cups chopped kale, wilted

½ cup grated mozzarella

Directions and Total Time: approx. 45 minutes

Preheat oven to 400 F. Line a pizza-baking pan with parchment paper. Whisk 6 eggs into a bowl and mix in in the provolone cheese and Italian seasoning. Spread the mixture on a pizza-baking pan and bake until golden, 15 minutes. Remove from oven and let cool for 2 minutes.

Fry bacon in a skillet over medium heat until brown and crispy, 5 minutes. Transfer to a plate. Spread tomato sauce on the crust, top with kale, mozzarella cheese, and mushrooms. Bake in the oven for 8 minutes. Crack the remaining 4 eggs on top, cover with bacon, and continue baking until the eggs set, 2-3 minutes. Serve sliced.

Per serving: Cal 893; Net Carbs 6g; Fat 67g; Protein 59g

Pork Medallions with Buttered Cabbage

Ingredients for 4 servings

1 ½ pork tenderloin, sliced into ½-inch medallions

6 tbsp butter

1 canon cabbage, shredded

Salt and black pepper to taste

1 celery, chopped

1 tbsp red curry powder

1 ¼ cups coconut cream

Directions and Total Time: approx. 45 minutes

Melt half of the butter in a skillet over medium heat and sauté cabbage for 10-15 minutes or until soft and slightly golden; reserve. Melt remaining butter in the skillet, add in celery, and sauté for 2 minutes. Add in the pork and fry until brown on the outside and cooked within 10 minutes. Season with salt and pepper and mix in curry and heat for 30 seconds. Stir in coconut cream and simmer for 5 minutes. Serve medallions with buttered cabbage.

Per serving: Cal 626; Net Carbs 3.9g; Fat 48g; Protein 43g

Mozzarella Baked Pork

Ingredients for 4 servings

4 boneless pork chops

Salt and black pepper to taste

1 cup golden flaxseed meal

1 large egg, beaten

1 cup tomato sauce

1 cup shredded mozzarella

Directions and Total Time: approx. 30 minutes

Preheat oven to 400 F. Season the pork with salt and pepper and coat the meat in the egg first, then in flaxseed. Place on a greased baking sheet. Pour tomato sauce over and sprinkle with mozzarella cheese. Bake for 15 minutes or until the cheese melts and pork cooks through. Serve.

Per serving: Cal 592; Net Carbs 2.7g; Fat 25g; Protein 62g

Cheesy Mushrooms & Bacon Lettuce Rolls

Ingredients for 4 servings

½ cup sliced cremini mushrooms

1 iceberg lettuce, leaves separated

8 bacon slices, chopped

2 tbsp olive oil

1 ½ lb ground pork

1 cup shredded cheddar

Directions and Total Time: approx. 30 minutes

In a skillet over medium heat, cook bacon until brown and crispy, about 5 minutes. Transfer to a paper-towel-lined plate. Heat the olive oil in the skillet and sauté the mushrooms for 5 minutes or until softened. Add in the ground pork and cook it until brown, 10 minutes, while breaking the lumps that form. Divide the pork between lettuce leaves, sprinkle with cheddar cheese, and top with bacon. Wrap and serve with mayonnaise.

Per serving: Cal 630; Net Carbs 0.5g; Fat 45g; Protein 52g

__Seafood__

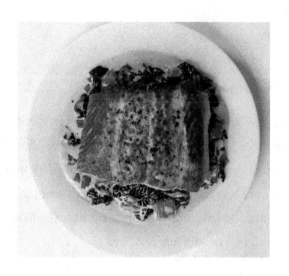

Cod & Cauliflower Parmesan Gratin

Ingredients for 4 servings

1 head cauliflower, cut into florets

2 cod fillets, cubed

3 white fish fillets, cubed

1 tbsp butter, melted

1 cup crème fraiche

¼ cup grated Parmesan

Grated Parmesan for topping

Directions and Total Time: approx. 40 minutes

Preheat oven to 400 F. Coat fish cubes and broccoli with butter. Spread on a greased baking dish. Mix crème fraiche with Parmesan cheese, pour, and smear the cream on the fish. Sprinkle with some more Parmesan cheese. Bake for 25-30 minutes. Let sit for 5 minutes and serve.

Per serving: Cal 354; Net Carbs 4g; Fat 17g; Protein 28g

Blackened Cod Tortillas with Slaw

Ingredients for 4 servings

2 tbsp olive oil

1 tsp chili powder

2 cod fillets

1 tsp paprika

4 zero carb tortillas

½ cup red cabbage, shredded

1 tbsp lemon juice

1 tsp apple cider vinegar

1 tbsp olive oil

Salt and black pepper to taste

Directions and Total Time: approx. 20 minutes

Season cod fillets with chili powder, paprika, salt, and pepper. Heat half of olive oil in a skillet over medium heat. Add cod and cook until blackened, about 6 minutes. Cut into strips. Divide the fish between the tortillas. Combine cabbage, lemon juice, vinegar, and remaining olive oil in a bowl; toss to combine. Add to the tortillas and serve.

Per serving: Cal 260; Net Carbs 3.5g; Fat 20g; Protein 14g

Hazelnut Cod Fillets

Ingredients for 2 servings

2 cod fillets

2 tbsp ghee

¼ cup roasted hazelnuts

A pinch of cayenne pepper

Directions and Total Time: approx. 30 minutes

Preheat your oven to 425 F. Line a baking dish with waxed paper. Melt the ghee and brush it over the fish. In a food processor, combine the rest of the ingredients. Coat the cod with the mixture. Transfer to the baking dish and bake for about 15 minutes. Serve warm.

Per serving: Cal 467; Net Carbs 2.8g; Fat 31g; Protein 40g

Nutty Sea Bass

Ingredients for 2 servings

2 sea bass fillets

2 tbsp butter

⅓ cup roasted hazelnuts

A pinch of cayenne pepper

Directions and Total Time: approx. 30 minutes

Preheat oven to 420 F. Line a baking dish with waxed paper. Melt butter and brush it over the fillets. In a food processor, combine the remaining ingredients. Coat the fish with the hazelnut mixture. Bake for 15 minutes. Serve.

Per serving: Cal 467; Net Carbs 2.8g; Fat 31g; Protein 40g

<u>Vegan and vegetarian</u>

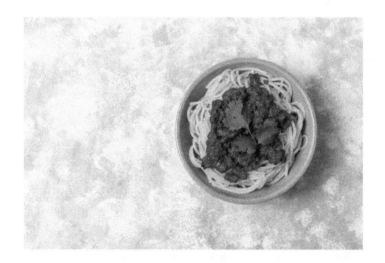

One-Skillet Green Pasta

Ingredients for 4 servings

1 cup shredded mozzarella cheese

1 cup grated Pecorino Romano cheese for topping

1 egg yolk

2 garlic cloves, minced

1 lemon, juiced

1 cup baby spinach

½ cup almond milk

1 avocado, pitted and peeled

1 tbsp olive oil

Salt to taste

Directions and Total Time: approx. 15 min + chilling time

Microwave mozzarella cheese for 2 minutes. Take out the bowl and allow cooling for 1 minute. Mix in egg yolk until well-combined. Lay a parchment paper on a flat surface, pour the cheese mixture on top and cover with another parchment paper. Flatten the dough into 1/8-inch thickness. Take off the parchment paper and cut the dough into thick fettuccine strands. Place in a bowl and refrigerate overnight. Bring 2 cups water to a boil in a saucepan and add the fettuccine. Cook for 1 minute and drain; set aside. In a blender, combine garlic, lemon juice, spinach, almond milk, avocado, olive oil, and salt. Process until smooth. Pour fettuccine into a bowl, top with sauce, and mix. Top with Pecorino Romano cheese and serve.

Per serving: Cal 290; Net Carbs 5g; Fats 19g; Protein 18g

Charred Asparagus with Creamy Sauce

Ingredients for 4 servings

½ lb asparagus, no hard stalks

Salt and chili pepper to taste

4 tbsp flax seed powder

½ cup coconut cream

1 cup butter, melted

⅓ cup mozzarella, grated

2 tbsp olive oil

Juice of half lemon

Directions and Total Time: approx. 12 minutes

Heat olive oil in a saucepan and roast the asparagus until lightly charred. Season with salt and set aside. Melt half of butter in a pan and stir until nutty and golden brown. Add in lemon juice and pour the mixture over the asparagus. In a safe microwave bowl, mix flax seed powder with ½ cup water and let sit for 5 minutes. Microwave flax egg 1-2 minutes, then pour into a blender. Add the remaining butter, mozzarella cheese, coconut cream, salt, and chili pepper. Puree until well combined and smooth. Serve.

Per serving: Cal 442; Net Carbs 5.4g; Fat 45g; Protein 5.9g

Speedy Custard Tart

Ingredients for 4 servings

¼ cup butter, cold

¼ cup almond flour

5 tbsp coconut flour

½ tsp salt

3 tbsp erythritol

1 ½ tsp vanilla extract

4 whole eggs

3 egg yolks

½ cup swerve sugar

1 tsp vanilla bean paste

1 ¼ cup almond milk

1 ¼ cup heavy cream

2 tbsp sugar-free maple syrup

¼ cup chopped almonds

Directions and Total Time: approx. 75 minutes

Preheat oven to 350 F. Grease a pie pan with cooking spray. In a bowl, mix almond flour, 3 tbsp coconut flour, and salt. Add in butter and mix with an electric mixer until crumbly. Add in erythritol and vanilla extract and mix. Pour in four eggs one after another while mixing until formed into a ball. Dust a clean flat surface with almond flour, unwrap the dough, and roll out the dough into a large rectangle, fit into the pie pan; prick the base of the crust. Bake until golden. Remove after and allow cooling.

In a bowl, whisk the remaining 2 eggs, egg yolks, swerve, vanilla, and remaining coconut flour. Put almond milk, heavy cream, and maple syrup into a pot and bring to a boil. Pour the mixture into the egg mix and whisk while pouring. Run batter through a fine strainer into a bowl and skim off any froth. Transfer the batter into the pie. Bake for 45 minutes. Garnish with almonds, slice, and serve.

Per serving: Cal 459; Net Carbs 1.2g, Fat 40g, Protein 12g

Mint Ice Cream

Ingredients for 4 servings

2 avocados, pitted

1 ¼ cups coconut cream

½ tsp vanilla extract

2 tbsp erythritol

2 tsp chopped mint leaves

Directions and Total Time: approx. 10 min+ chilling time

Into a blender, spoon avocado pulps, pour in coconut cream, vanilla extract, erythritol, and mint leaves. Process until smooth. Pour the mixture into your ice cream maker and freeze according to the manufacturer's instructions. When ready, remove, and scoop the ice cream into bowls.

Per serving: Cal 370; Net Carbs 4g; Fat 38g; Protein 4g

Sweet Onion & Goat Cheese Pizza

Ingredients for 4 servings

2 cups grated mozzarella

2 tbsp cream cheese, softened

2 large eggs, beaten

⅓ cup almond flour

1 tsp dried Italian seasoning

2 tbsp butter

2 red onions, thinly sliced

1 cup crumbled goat cheese

1 tbs almond milk

1 cup curly endive, chopped

Directions and Total Time: approx. 35 minutes

Preheat oven to 390 F. Line a round pizza pan with parchment paper. Microwave the mozzarella and cream cheeses for 1 minute. Remove and mix in eggs, almond flour, and Italian seasoning. Spread the dough on the pizza pan and bake for 6 minutes. Melt butter in a skillet and stir in onions, salt, and pepper and cook on low heat with frequent stirring until caramelized, 15-20 minutes. In a bowl, mix goat cheese with almond milk and spread on the crust. Top with the caramelized onions. Bake for 10 minutes. Scatter curly endive on top, slice, and serve.

Per serving: Cal 317; Net Carbs 3g; Fats 20g; Protein 28g

Spinach-Olive Pizza

Ingredients for 4 servings

1 cup grated mozzarella

½ cup almond flour

¼ tsp salt

2 tbsp ground psyllium husk

1 tbsp olive oil

1 cup lukewarm water

½ cup tomato sauce

½ cup baby spinach

1 tsp dried oregano

3 tbsp sliced black olives

Directions and Total Time: approx. 40 minutes

Preheat oven to 390 F. Line a baking sheet with parchment paper. In a bowl, mix almond flour, salt, psyllium husk, olive oil, and water until dough forms. Spread the mixture on the sheet and bake for 10 minutes. Remove the crust and spread the tomato sauce on top. Add spinach, mozzarella cheese, oregano, and olives. Bake for 15 minutes. Take out of the oven, slice, and serve warm.

Per serving: Cal 195; Net Carbs 1.8g; Fats 8g; Protein 11g

Tofu Nuggets with Cilantro Dip

Ingredients for 4 servings

1 lime, ½ juiced and ½ cut into wedges

1 ½ cups olive oil

28 oz tofu, pressed and cubed

1 egg, lightly beaten

1 cup golden flaxseed meal

1 ripe avocado, chopped

½ tbsp chopped cilantro

Salt and black pepper to taste

½ tbsp olive oil

Directions and Total Time: approx. 25 minutes

Heat olive oil in a deep skillet. Coat tofu cubes in the egg and then in the flaxseed meal. Fry until golden brown. Transfer to a plate. Place avocado, cilantro, salt, pepper, and lime juice in a blender; puree until smooth. Spoon into a bowl, add tofu nuggets, and lime wedges to serve.

Per serving: Cal 665; Net Carbs 6.2g, Fat 54g, Protein 32g

Snacks and side dish

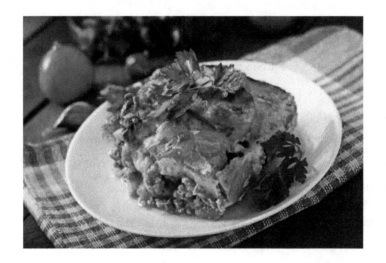

Crunchy Rutabaga Puffs

Ingredients for 4 servings

1 rutabaga, peeled and diced

2 tbsp melted butter

½ oz goat cheese, crumbled

¼ cup ground pork rinds

Directions and Total Time: approx. 35 minutes

Preheat oven to 400 F. Spread rutabaga on a baking sheet and drizzle with the butter. Bake until tender, 15 minutes. Transfer to a bowl. Allow cooling and add in goat cheese. Using a fork, mash and mix the ingredients. Pour the pork rinds onto a plate. Mold 1-inch balls out of the rutabaga mixture and roll properly in the rinds while pressing gently to stick. Place in the same baking sheet and bake for 10 minutes until golden. Serve.

Per serving: Cal 129; Net Carbs 5.9g; Fat 8g; Protein 3g

Crispy Pancetta & Butternut Squash Roast

Ingredients for 4 servings

2 butternut squash, cubed

1 tsp turmeric powder

½ tsp garlic powder

8 pancetta slices, chopped

2 tbsp olive oil

1 tbsp chopped cilantro,

Directions and Total Time: approx. 30 minutes

Preheat oven to 425 F. In a bowl, add butternut squash, turmeric, garlic powder, pancetta, and olive oil. Toss until well-coated. Spread the mixture onto a greased baking sheet and roast for 10-15 minutes. Transfer the veggies to a bowl and garnish with cilantro to serve.

Per serving: Cal 148; Net Carbs 6.4g; Fat 10g; Protein 6g

Paprika & Dill Deviled Eggs

Ingredients for 4 servings

1 tsp dill, chopped

8 large eggs

3 cups water

3 tbsp sriracha sauce

4 tbsp mayonnaise

¼ tsp sweet paprika

Directions and Total Time: approx. 20 minutes

Bring eggs to a boil in salted water and cook for 10 minutes. Transfer to an ice water bath, let cool completely and peel the shells. Slice the eggs in half lengthwise and empty the yolks into a bowl. Smash with a fork and mix in sriracha sauce, mayonnaise, and paprika until smooth. Spoon filling into a piping bag and fill the egg whites to be slightly above the brim. Garnish with dill and serve.

Per serving: Cal 195; Net Carbs 1g; Fat 19g; Protein 4g

Simple Stuffed Eggs with Mayonnaise

Ingredients for 6 servings

6 eggs

1 tbsp green tabasco

¼ cup mayonnaise

2 tbsp black olives, sliced

Directions and Total Time: approx. 30 minutes

Place eggs in a salted boiling water and cook for 10 minutes. Remove the eggs to an ice bath and let cool. Peel and slice in half lengthwise. Scoop out the yolks to a bowl; mash with a fork. Whisk together the tabasco, mayonnaise, and mashed yolks in a bowl. Spoon this mixture into egg whites. Garnish with olives and serve.

Per serving: Cal 178; Net Carbs: 5g; Fat: 17g; Protein: 6g

Cheesy Pork Rind Bread

Ingredients for 4 servings

¼ cup grated Pecorino Romano cheese

8 oz cream cheese

2 cups grated mozzarella

1 tbsp baking powder

1 cup crushed pork rinds

3 large eggs

1 tbsp Italian mixed herbs

Directions and Total Time: approx. 30 minutes

Preheat oven to 375 F. Line a baking sheet with parchment paper. Microwave cream and mozzarella cheeses for 1 minute or until melted. Whisk in baking powder, pork rinds, eggs, Pecorino Romano cheese, and Italian mixed herbs. Spread the mixture in the baking sheet and bake for 20 minutes until lightly brown. Let cool, slice, and serve.

Per serving: Cal 437; Net Carbs 3.2g; Fat 23g; Protein 32g

Baked Spicy Eggplants

Ingredients for 4 servings

2 large eggplants

2 tbsp butter

1 tsp red chili flakes

4 oz raw ground almonds

Directions and Total Time: approx. 30 minutes

Preheat oven to 400 F. Cut off the head of the eggplants and slice the body into rounds. Arrange on a parchment paper-lined baking sheet. Drop thin slices of butter on each eggplant slice, sprinkle with chili flakes, and bake for 20 minutes. Slide out and sprinkle with almonds. Roast further for 5 minutes. Serve with arugula salad.

Per serving: Cal 230; Net Carbs 4g; Fat 16g; Protein 14g

Prosciutto Appetizer with Blackberries

Ingredients for 4 servings

4 zero carb bread slices

¾ cup balsamic vinegar

1 tbsp erythritol

1 cup fresh blackberries

1 cup crumbled goat cheese

¼ tsp dry Italian seasoning

1 tbsp almond milk

4 thin prosciutto slices

Directions and Total Time: approx. 25 minutes

Cut the bread into 3 pieces each and arrange on a baking sheet. Place under the broiler and toast for 1-2 minutes on each side or until golden brown; set aside. In a saucepan, add balsamic vinegar and stir in erythritol until dissolved. Boil the mixture over medium heat until reduced by half, 5 minutes. Turn the heat off and carefully stir in the blackberries. Make sure they do not break open. Set aside.In a bowl, add goat cheese, Italian seasoning, and almond milk. Mix until smooth. Brush one side of the toasted bread with the balsamic reduction and top with the cheese mixture. Cut each prosciutto slice into 3 pieces and place on the bread. Top with some of the whole blackberries from the balsamic mixture. Serve immediately.

Per serving: Cal 175; Net Carbs 8.7g; Fat 7g; Protein 18g

Dessert

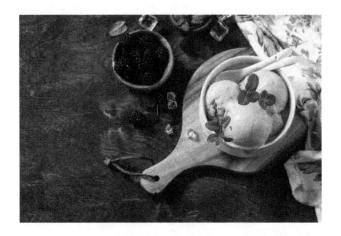

Choco-Coffee Cake

Ingredients for 4 servings

3 tbsp golden flaxseed meal, ground

1 tbsp melted butter

1 cup almond flour

2 tbsp coconut flour

1 tsp baking powder

¼ cup cocoa powder

¼ tsp salt

½ tsp espresso powder

1/3-½ cup coconut sugar

¼ tsp xanthan gum

¼ cup organic coconut oil

2 tbsp heavy cream

2 eggs

Directions and Total Time: approx. 30 minutes

Preheat oven to 400 F. Grease a springform pan with melted butter. In a bowl, mix almond flour, flaxseed meal, coconut flour, baking powder, cocoa powder, salt, espresso, coconut sugar, and xanthan gum. In another bowl, whisk coconut oil, heavy cream, and eggs. Combine both mixtures until smooth batter forms. Pour the batter into the pan and bake until a toothpick comes out clean, 20 minutes. Transfer to a wire rack, let cool, slice, and serve.

Chocolate Snowball Cookies

Ingredients for 4 servings

¼ cup swerve confectioner's sugar

1 cup butter, softened

½ cups erythritol, divided

2 cups almond flour

2 tsp cocoa powder

1 tsp vanilla extract

1 cup pecans, finely chopped

½ tsp salt

2 tbsp water

Directions and Total Time: approx. 35 min + chilling time

Preheat oven to 325 F. Line a baking sheet with parchment paper. In a bowl, using a hand mixer, cream the butter and erythritol. Fold in almond flour, cocoa powder, vanilla, pecans, salt, and water. Mold 1 tbsp cookie dough from the mixture and place on the sheet. Chill for 1 hour. Transfer to the sheet and bake for 25 minutes or until the cookies look dry and colorless. Remove them from the oven to cool for 10 minutes. Sprinkle with swerve to serve.

Per serving: Cal 584; Net Carbs 3.7g; Fat 61g; Protein 3g

Peanut Butter Almond Cookies

Ingredients for 4 servings

½ cup peanut butter, softened

2 cups almond flour

½ tsp baking soda

1 cup xylitol

A pinch of salt

2 tbsp xylitol

1 tsp ground cardamom pods

Directions and Total Time: approx. 25 minutes

Combine peanut butter, almond flour, baking soda, ¾ cup of xylitol, and salt in a bowl. Form balls out of the mixture and flatten them. Combine cardamom and remaining xylitol. Dip in the biscuits and arrange them on a lined cookie sheet. Cook in the oven for 15-20 minutes at 350 F.

Per serving: Cal 96; Net Carbs 7.4g; Fat 6.1g; Protein 2.4g

Chocolate Cake with Raspberry Frosting

Ingredients for 6 servings

2 cups blanched almond flour

1 cup erythritol

½ cup cocoa powder

1 tsp baking powder

½ cup butter, softened

1 tsp vanilla extract

2 eggs

1 cup almond milk

For the frosting:

8 oz cream cheese, softened

½ cup butter, softened

1 cup fresh raspberries, mashed

3 tbsp cocoa powder

2 tbsp heavy whipping cream

1/3 cup powdered erythritol

1 tsp vanilla extract

Directions and Total Time: approx. 40 minutes

Preheat oven to 350 degrees. In a bowl, mix almond flour, erythritol, cocoa powder, and baking powder until fully combined. Mix in butter and vanilla. Crack open the eggs into the bowl and whisk until completely combined; stir in

103

almond milk. Prepare three 6-inch round cake pans and generously grease with butter. Divide the batter into the 3 cake pans. Place all the pans in the oven and bake for 25 minutes or until the cakes set. Remove them to a wire rack. In a bowl, whip cream cheese, butter, raspberries, cocoa powder, heavy cream, erythritol, and vanilla extract until smooth. To assemble: place the first cake on a flat surface and spread ⅓ of the frosting over top. Place second cake layer, add and smoothen the frosting, and then do the same for the last cake. Slice and serve immediately.

Per serving: Cal 546; Net Carbs 8.4g; Fat 46g; Protein 9g

Matcha Fat Bombs

Ingredients for 4 servings

½ cup coconut oil

1 tbsp vanilla extract

½ cup almond butter

4 tbsp matcha powder powder

½ cup xylitol

Directions and Total Time: approx. 3 min + cooling time

Melt almond butter and coconut oil in a saucepan over low heat, stirring until properly melted and mixed. Mix in matcha powder and xylitol until combined. Pour into muffin moulds and refrigerate for 3 hours to harden.

Per serving: Cal 436; Net Carbs 3.1g; Fat 44.6g; Protein 6g

Coffee Balls

Ingredients for 6 servings

1 ½ cups mascarpone cheese

½ cup melted ghee

3 tbsp cocoa powder

¼ cup erythritol

6 tbsp brewed coffee

Directions and Total Time: approx. 3 min + cooling time

Whisk mascarpone, ghee, cocoa powder, erythritol, and coffee with a hand mixer until creamy and fluffy, about 1 minute. Fill in muffin tins and freeze for 3 hours until firm.

Per serving: Cal 145; Net Carbs 2g; Fat 14g; Protein 4g

Classic Zucchini Cake

Ingredients for 4 servings

4 egg

4 tbsp butter, melted

½ tsp vanilla extract

¼ cup sugar-free maple syrup

1 ½ cups almond flour

½ cup swerve sugar

1 ½ tsp baking powder

¼ tsp baking soda

½ tsp salt

1 ¼ tsp cinnamon

½ tsp nutmeg

⅛ tsp ground cloves

1 cup grated zucchinis

Directions and Total Time: approx. 30 minutes

Preheat oven to 400 F. Grease a cake pan with melted butter. In a bowl, beat the eggs, butter, most of the maple syrup, and vanilla extract until smooth. In another bowl, mix almond flour, swerve sugar, baking powder, baking soda, salt, cinnamon, and ground cloves. Combine both mixtures until smooth, fold in the zucchinis and pour the batter into the cake pan. Bake for 25 minutes or until a toothpick inserted comes out clean. Transfer to a wire rack, let cool, and drizzle with the remaining maple syrup all over. Slice and serve.

Per serving: Cal 235; Net Carbs 6.3g; Fat 21g; Protein 9g

Keto Caramel Shortbread Cookies

Ingredients for 8 servings

¼ cup sugar-free caramel sauce

2 cups butter

1 ½ cups swerve brown sugar

3 cups almond flour

1 cup chopped dark chocolate

Sea salt flakes

Directions and Total Time: approx. 30 minutes

Preheat oven to 350 F. Line a baking sheet with parchment paper. In a bowl, using an electric mixer, whisk butter, swerve, and caramel sauce. Mix in flour and chocolate until well combined. Using a scoop, arrange 1 ½ tbsp of the batter onto the sheet at 2-inch intervals and sprinkle salt flakes on top. Bake for 15 minutes until lightly golden.

Per serving: Cal 410; Net Carbs 0.6g; Fat 43g; Protein 5g

Blueberry Tart

Ingredients for 4 servings

4 eggs

2 tsp coconut oil

2 cups blueberries

1 cup coconut milk

1 cup almond flour

¼ cup sweetener

½ tsp vanilla powder

1 tbsp powdered sweetener

A pinch of salt

Directions and Total Time: approx. 45 minutes

Preheat oven to 350 F. Place all ingredients except coconut oil, berries, and powdered sweetener in a blender, and blend until smooth. Gently fold in the berries. Pour the mixture into a greased dish and bake for 35 minutes. Sprinkle with powdered sweetener.

Per serving: Cal 355; Net Carbs 6.9g; Fat 14g; Protein 12g

CPSIA information can be obtained
at www.ICGtesting.com
Printed in the USA
BVHW050156060321
601818BV00006B/794